The Comp Alkaline Diet For Beginners

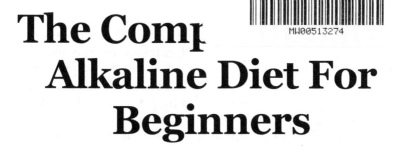

Clean Your Body, Reverse Diabetes, Reset Inflammation, Lose Weight and Boost Energy by eating PH Basic foods

2-Week Meal Plan Menu Included

By

Anna Lor

Table of Content

Introduction

In this book, we will discuss the recommendations and all about alkaline diets. We must first find out what the alkaline diet is. An alkaline diet is known as the PHenomenon miracle, PH equilibrium diet and acidic diet. It is based on the idea that anything you consume will either cause your body to develop acid or alkaline. This can be awful to figure out what is right (alkaline) and what is wrong (acidic) for anyone beginning this diet. That is why I wanted to compile and thus explain some of the uncertainties in the alkaline diet.

There are also recommendations for alkaline diets. The underlying principle is that some chemicals are harmful to the body than others. One of the proposals for the alkaline diet is to try 75-80 percent alkaline. This means that 75-80% of your diet comes from the alkaline food map. However, some foods are known to be more acidic than others. Here's a list of foods that can be thought to be extremely acidic according to the alkaline diet: sweeteners (equal, sweet and low, sweet nutrients and some of them aspartame), beer, salts, jelly, ice cream, meat, lobster, fried food, refined from wells and soft drinks. Here's a fun fact that cola has 2.5 PH. It's very acidic. You need to drink like 32 glasses of water to neutralize the can of cola.

There are certain foods on the other side of the spectrum that are considered to be highly alkaline, and that increase the alkalinity of the body when ingested.

The alkaline diet recommendations suggest medications which are also highly acidic. Think of all those who take some kind of medicine to relieve their acid reflux. They don't know that their temporary solution causes them significant problems in the long run. Many other alkaline diets are available. The more you eat, the better you're going to feel. Many times, when people move to the alkaline diet, they experience detoxification. The guidelines for the alkaline diet suggest that you spend a few weeks detoxifying your body and allowing it to adjust to this entirely new way of eating.

Chapter 1: What Is an Alkaline Diet?

An alkaline diet consists of a meal plan empHasizing the primary source of food, fresh vegetables, tubers, fruit, roots, nuts and legumes. This kind of food plan has become very popular as we understand the excellent health benefits of specific raw foods.

A high intake of alkaline food helps to control acid concentrations in the body. With a PH strip in the morning, you can easily verify your PH. PH levels below seven are known to be acidic and hazardous to your wellbeing. PH levels between 7.3 and 7.45 are considered to be optimal for good health.

Then why are you really supposed to think about that? Alkalization is so essential because the body cells perform better in a moderately alkaline environment, whereas harmful organisms such as cancers develop in an acidic environment. Studies show that cancer cells are killed within an hour when a body hits 8.0 PH equilibrium!

The most critical cause of osteoporosis? You guessed high levels of acidity in the body are typically caused by too much meat.

Foods that contribute to an acidic body climate include milk, meats, sucrose snacks, caffeine, soda and processed food. These are the foods that some people consume every day.

The best way to ensure a balanced, non-acidic diet is to get the majority of your food from fresh, living organic foods. Just spend at least two weeks eating high alkaline food and then slowly start adding other food, and immediately you will see what food works for you and which foods work against you. This form of food is also called a detox diet because acidic toxins are washed out of the body.

Avocado, celery, salad, dandelion, sprout radishes, colt, cucumber, barley grass, alfalfa grass, tomato, beans and much more are healthy food for your detox.

Beer, eggs, pistachios, cheese, ketchup, veal, pork, white bread, spirits, sea fish, and artificial sweeteners to mention only a few are acidic foods which need to be avoided.

Most people appreciate a miraculous difference in how they look and feel on this form of diet after only a few days. Raw diets are good because it's fast and simple to prepare; not to mention, there's an endless variety of food that you can enjoy in this type of diet.

In order to understand the significance of the Alkaline Diet and the effect of certain foods on our bodies, it is essential to understand the fundamentals of the food we consume.

The Alkaline Diet fundamentally separates food into two classes- alkaline and acidic. In order to explain further the importance of alkaline and acidic terms, the ash left in the food once eaten by your body is represented. So essentially when we speak about acid or alkaline the simple acid ash or alkaline ash that is left when the food is digested is referred to.

It can be a little challenging to distinguish what is the food because although lemons are considered acidic in nature, they leave a very alkaline ash in the body after they are digested.

So, when in terms of alkaline diet, it's referred to as acidic, we don't mention the properties of the food as such, but rather the simple ash it leaves on the body, where foods that leave alkaline ash are the favored option.

Foods with acidic qualities but strongly alkaline ash. Foods considered acidic but extremely alkaline in our bodies are:

- Limes
- Grapefruit
- Tomatoes
- Lemons

That means they're perfect for you!

Alkaline foodstuffs

Most of the plants are considered alkaline, and the green ones are especially good for you.

The vegetable list (but not limited to) includes:

- Beets
- Avocado
- Carrots

- Cauliflower

- Green beans

- Corn

- Garlic

- Cucumber

- Peas

- Peppers pumpkins

- Onions

The fruits are known to be mildly acidic, and they should be limited to 20% of the remainder of the Alkadi, 80% of which are vegetables.

Fruit considered alkaline are:

- Coconut

- Bananas

- Watermelon

The remaining fruits are considered acidic.

Fruits falling within the acidic spectrum, but not restricted to:

- Apricots

- Apples

- Dates

- Grapes

- Figs

- Mangos

- Papayas

- Oranges

- Nectarines

- Peaches

- Pineapples
- Pears

Foods are known to be strongly acidic include:

- Lamb
- Beef
- Wine
- Crayfish
- Crab
- Cold cuts
- Whole eggs

For optimal health and resources, the alkaline diet advises that your consumption should include 80% alkaline foods and 20% acidic foods. It is essential to keep your food healthy, as leaning too heavily can affect your health. You get sick and vice versa if your body is too alkaline, so one needs common sense when it comes to preparing daily meals.

Alkaline Diet - How Does It Help?

This diet has recently gained popularity among diet and nutrition experts and writers. The effectiveness of the alkaline diet is still being debated since there is no clear proof that alkaline diets can minimize those diseases.

This is because these foods have been digested, ingested and metabolized and released alkaline. On the other hand, after processes, meat, milk, salts and cereals contain acid. Food is graded as acid-producing or alkaline-producing food based on PH (hydrogen-energy) values with an acidic PH of 0 to 6, an alkaline PH of 8 to 14 and a water-neutral PH of 7. Therefore, the alkaline diet refers to the diet in which more alkaline food is made.

Alkaline Diet

Our blood has a slightly alkaline PH between 7.35 and 7.45. The alkaline diet is based on our blood PH, and any high acid-producing diet would disorder the balance. The acidity of the food leads to the depletion of essential minerals such as potassium, magnesium, calcium and sodium whenever the organism seeks to revitalize the balance of PH in its blood. Disequilibrium can make people vulnerable to disease.

Sadly, Western diets contain more acid and eat a few fresh vegetables and fruits. The norm of the Western diet has changed considerably as a result of the introduction of the alkaline diet.

Some dieticians claim that acidic diets can cause some chronic disease and the following symptoms, such as:

- Nervousness, anxiety,

- Headache

- Lethargic

- Recurrent cold and flu and increased development of mucosa

- Vaginal cysts, brain cysts, polycystic ovaries

Although most believe that the above conditions are the consequence of acid production and fruit and vegetable consumption is beneficial for health, some Physicians claim that an acid-producing diet does not cause chronic diseases. Furthermore, there is evidence that alkaline diets help to protect against the development of calcium kidney stones, osteoporosis and muscle wastage linked to age.

Balance Diet

While alkaline diets are favored, extreme diets (eat all alkaline-producing foods) are not recommended. It is better to aim for healthy intermediate soil for both food forms. Only remember to take note of the above indicators and consult a doctor before attempting a new diet.

Benefits of Alkaline Diet for Diabetics

Body style and diet alkaline

To a certain extent, the human body is alkaline by nature. By keeping it alkaline, we allow it to run ideally. Despite this, millions of metabolism reactions produce acidic waste as final products. If we eat too many acid-producing foods and not adequate alkaline-forming foods, it makes body acid intoxication worse. A disease known as acidosis develops over time if we encourage the build-up of these acid wastes through the body.

Acidosis will eventually weaken our essential functions if we do not take remedial steps quickly. Acidosis is actually one of the leading causes of human aging. It makes our bodies extremely vulnerable to a variety of lethal chronic diseases, including diabetes, cancer, arthritis and cardiovascular diseases.

Therefore, the greatest challenge for us humans to face in order to protect our lives is actually to find the best way to reduce the production and optimize the removal of body acid waste. Our body requires a balanced lifestyle to prevent acidosis and age-related diseases and to continue to function at the highest possible level. This lifestyle should include daily workouts, healthy diet, clean Physical environments and living conditions that provide the lowest possible stress. A balanced lifestyle helps our body to achieve the lowest possible acid waste content.

The alkaline diet seems to suit the body's best design. The main explanation is that it contributes to the neutralization of acid waste and allows it to be wasted from the body. People should accept alkaline diets as general dietary limits to be respected by humans. People with special health conditions and medical diets could better accommodate these diets to alkaline diet limits.

Alkaline Diabetic Benefits

The miracle alkaline diet will improve people with diabetes' overall health. As for other people, alkaline diets help improve their physiology, metabolism and immune systems. This diet allows diabetics to regulate their blood sugar better. It would also help not only to minimize their weight gain and the risks of cardiovascular disease but also to maintain a lower level of cholesterol.

Indeed, the alkaline diet allows better treatment of diabetes and thereby enables diabetics to prevent degenerative symptoms more quickly. Thus, by adopting an alkaline diet in spite of their health, diabetics will simultaneously live better and boost their life expectancy considerably.

Acid-Alkaline Diet Map Diabetics

In general, people who choose to adopt an alkaline diet need to use the 'acid-alkaline food map' for their everyday food. A new

'Diabetics Acid-Alkaline Food Map' has been released. Using this map, diabetics should comply both with the alkaline diet rule and with the glycemic index rule.

The alkaline diet rules set general guidelines on nutrition. According to this diet schedule, our daily dietary intake must include no less than 80% of alkaline foods and no more than 20% of acidified foods. The diet additionally shows that the more alkaline a foodstuff is, the stronger it is and the more acidifying a foodstuff is, the worse for the human body.

With regard to the glycemic index law, foods are classified into four critical categories as regards their ability to increase the sugar content. The glycemic index GI of 0 to 100 now tests this ability.

- Food containing almost no glucose, and therefore having an insignificant glycemic index (GI~0), can be taken freely by diabetics.

- Low glycemic carbohydrate food (GI 55 or less); diabetes-related people should be careful to eat these products.

- Foodstuffs that have high-glycemic-index carbohydrates (GI56 or higher); diabetics should, as far as possible, exclude them from their diets.

- Processed food; diabetics shall consult manufacturers' labels for their glycemic index values.

Top Positive and Top Worst Diabetic Diets

The 'Diabetics Acid-Alkaline Diet Map' for people with diabetes divides diet into six groups. The following list ranges from the best to the worst foods.

1. **Alkalizing GI~0 food products. They are one of the best foods. Diabetics can eat free of charge.**

Asparagus, peanut, broccoli, lettuce, vegetable juices, chives, carob, squash, zucchini, okra, cauliflower, garlic/onions, beets, green bean, cold, limes, raw spinach, from herbal teas, stevia, lemon water, tea ginger, green tea, canola oil, olive oil, flax-seed oil.

2. Alkalization of foodstuffs having a GI of 55 or less. Diabetes patients should take them moderately due to their glycemic index.

Barley grass, sweet pumpkin, fresh maize, carrots, olives, tomatoes, peas/soya, bananas, mangoes, cherries, oranges, pears, kiwi, peaches, Popova, apples, fruit berries, wild roast, Brazil nut, chestnuts, coconut, lentils, quinoa, soy milk, breast milk, goat milk, raw honey, whey.

3. Acidifying GI~0 foods. Diabetics should take their acid-producing character carefully.

Fried spinach, shellfish, pork, oysters, lamb, cold-water fish, beef, poison, buttermilk, eggs, butter, cottage chocolate, maize oils, chocolate, margarine, wine, sunflower oil, beers, tea, coffee, mayonnaise, vinegar, mustard, artificial sweeteners.

4. Food acidification with GIs of 55 or less. Given the acid-forming and glycemic index of both, people with diabetes would need to eat them with caution.

Cranberries, sour cherries, plums, plums, brown rice, sprouted wheat bread, maize, peanuts, oats/rye, ice cream, whole-grain wheat/rye bread, walnuts, pasta, pistachios, pecans, cashews, sunflower seeds, yogurt, sesame, cream, sausage, custard, raw milk, homogenized milk, chocolate.

5. Foods are creating alkaline with a GI of 56 or higher. These goods are one of the worst foods for diabetics due to their high glycemic index. People with diabetes, therefore, ought to stop them.

Turnip, tofu, mackerel syrup, skin potato, figs, grapes / raisins, melons, dates, watermelon, raw sugar, beetroot, maple syrup, amaranth, millet.

6. Foods that contain acid with a GI of 56 or more. These papers are too acidic and carbohydrate too strongly glycemic. They are the worst food for diabetics. Diabetes sufferers must then wholly cut them off from their meals.

White bread refined sweet sugar, buckwheat, white rice, pumpkin, spelt, white sugar, white sugar, soft beverages.

The Alkaline Diet Myth

The alkaline diet is often referred to as the acid-alkaline diet or the ash diet. It is based on the premise that the food you consume leaves a trace behind the "ash" after it is metabolized. This ash may be either alkaline or acidic.

The advocates of this diet believe that specific foods, including urine and blood, can influence the acidity and alkalinity of body fluids. If you eat acidic ash foods, they make the body acidic. If you consume food with alkaline ash, it alkalizes the body.

Acid ash is meant to make you vulnerable to diseases such as osteoporosis, cancer and the wasting of muscles, whereas alkaline ash is known as healthy. In order to ensure you remain alkaline, you can keep track of your urine with functional PH test strips.

Diary arguments like this are very compelling for those who do not entirely understand human physiology and are not nutrition experts. But is it really true? The following will reverse this misconception and explain some uncertainty about the alkaline diet.

But first, the significance of the PH value must be understood.

Simply put, the PH value is an indicator of how acidic or alkaline is.

The PH value is between 0 and 14.

- Acidic 0-7

- Seven is neutral

- Alkaline 7-14

The stomach is, for instance, filled with strongly acidic hydrochloric acid, with a PH value of 2 to 3.5. The acidity helps to destroy germs and break food down.

The human blood, on the other hand, is often slightly alkaline at a PH of between 7.35 and 7.45. Usually, the body has many important (discussed later) mechanisms for preserving blood PH in this range. It is really severe and can be fatal to fall out.

Food effects on urine and blood PH

Foods leave an acid or alkaline ash behind them. Acid ash contains Phosphate and Sulphur. Calcium, potassium and magnesium are present in alkaline ash.

Acidic, or alkaline are considered in certain food classes.

- Acidic: fish, foods, eggs, grains, milk products, alcohol.
- Fats, sugars and starches are neutral.
- Alkaline: fruit, nuts, vegetables, herbs and vegetables. PH urine

You eat foods that change your urine's PH. If you get a green breakfast smoothie, the urine would be more alkaline in a few hours than if you had bacon and eggs.

For people on an alkaline diet, urine PH can be tracked very quickly and can provide immediate satisfaction. The urine PH is sadly neither a good indicator of the body's total PH nor a good indicator of general health.

The PH of the blood

The food you consume doesn't affect your blood PH. If you consume anything like acid ash, it will quickly neutralize the acids you generate with bicarbonate ions in the blood. This reaction produces carbon dioxide that is excreted through the lungs and salts excreted in the urine through the kidneys.

The kidney creates fresh bicarbonate ions during the excretion process that are returned to the blood to replace the previously used bicarbonate to neutralize the acid. This provides a sustainable cycle in which the body can maintain a tight PH of the blood.

Therefore, though your kidney functions normally, your blood's PH will not be affected by acidic or alkaline foods you consume. It is not true that consuming alkaline foods can make the body or blood PH alkaline.

Diet of Acidity and Cancer

Many who support an alkaline diet claim it will cure cancer because cancer is only able to increase in an acidic environment. Cancer cells cannot develop but die by consuming an alkaline diet.

This is a really inaccurate theory. Cancer can grow correctly in an alkaline climate. Cancer actually develops in normal body tissue with a slightly alkaline PH of 7.4. This is verified by several studies in the efficient growth of cancer cells in an alkaline environment.

However, acidity raises cancer cells faster. When a tumor begins to form, acidity is produced by breaking down glucose and reducing circulation. It is therefore not the acidic environment which causes cancer, but the acidic environment that causes cancer.

A research of the National Cancer Institute using vitamin C (ascorbic acid) for cancer is even more critical. They found that ascorbic acid effectively destroyed cancer cells without damaging normal cells by taking intravenously Pharmacological doses. This is another example of the susceptibility of cancer cells to acidity rather than alkalinity.

In short, no scientific link exists between acidic diet and cancer. In acidic and alkaline environments, cancer cells can expand.

Osteoporosis and Acidic Diet

Osteoporosis is a progressive bone condition with a decline of bone mineral content that causes a lower bone density and strength and a greater risk of a broken bone.

Alkaline diet advocates claim that the body uses alkaline minerals like calcium in its bones to neutralize the acids of the acidic diet to maintain a clear blood PH. As discussed above, this is not true at all. The blood PH is managed by the kidneys and the respiratory system, not the bones.

In fact, many studies proved that increasing the intake of animal protein is beneficial for the metabolism of bones because it increases calcium retention and activates IGF-1 (insulin-like growth factor-1). Therefore, the proof does not support the theory that an acidic diet induces bone loss.

Acidic Diet and Wasting of Muscle

Advocates of the alkaline diet assume that the kidneys can steal amino acids from muscle tissue (protein building blocks) in order to remove the acid overload caused by acidic diet, contributing to muscle failure. The mechanism proposed is similar to that which causes osteoporosis.

Blood PH is regulated by the kidneys and lungs, not the muscles, as discussed. Acidic foods such as meats, milk and eggs also do not cause muscle failure. Indeed, they are complete dietary proteins that aid muscle repair and prevent loss of muscle.

What have our ancestors been eating?

There have been studies examining whether our pre-farming ancestors consumed net acidic or net alkaline diets. Somewhat surprisingly, they found that roughly half of the hunter collectors consumed net acid-forming diets, while the other half consumed net alkalines.

Acid-forming diets were more prevalent as people went north of the equator. The less environmentally conscious, the more animal proteins you consumed. Their diet became more alkaline in tropical conditions in which fruits and vegetables were plentiful.

The hypothesis that acidic or protein-rich diets cause diseases such as cancer, osteoporosis and Muscle loss from an evolutionary perspective is not true. Half the hunter collectors had a net acid-forming diet, but there was no evidence of such degenerative diseases.

It should be remembered that no single-sized diet works for everyone, so Metabolic Typing is so helpful in deciding your ideal diet. Because of our genetic variances, certain people benefit from acidic, alkaline, and intermediate diets. So the saying: one man's food can be another man's poison.

Many people who have adjusted to an alkaline diet are seeing significant changes in wellbeing. Nevertheless, note that other motives might be at work:

- Most of us don't eat enough fruit and vegetables. Just 9% of Americans consume enough vegetables, and 13% eat enough fruits, according to the Centre for Disease and Prevention. You naturally eat more vegetables and fruit when you turn to an alkaline diet. After all, they are highly rich for good health with Phytochemicals, antioxidants and fiber. If you consume more vegetables and fruit, you probably will consume less processed foods.

- Less milk and eggs would be helpful for those that are lactose intolerant or egg-allergic, which is popular in the general population.

- Less grain intake can help those who are gluten sensitive or who have an autoimmune or leaky intestinal disorder.

Alkaline Water

Many people assume that consuming alkaline water (PH 9.5 vs plain water PH 7.0) is better since the alkaline diet is equally reasoned. It's not real, anyway. Too alkaline water can harm your health and lead to nutritional imbalance.

If you only drink alkaline water, it will neutralize your stomach acid and increase your stomach alkalinity. Over time, this reduces the ability to digest food and consume minerals and nutrients. With less acidity in the stomach, bacteria and parasites may also be opened to access the small gut.

Basically, alkaline water isn't the key to good health. Don't be fooled by marketing jokes. Invest instead in a successful home water filtration system. Clean, filtered water is always the body's best water.

Chapter2: 2 Weeks Meal Plan

If your healthy habits have gone wrong, this easy clean-up meal plan will help you to re-establish the eating habits that help you feel the best. In the course of this 14-day diet plan, some nutritious foods you cook from scratch and those that you can purchase from the shop will be filled.

If you're new to clean food, the idea is easy, and a meal plan will make it even easier to understand (or simply use for inspiration). Clean-eating is a perfect way to improve your food sources, while at the same time restricting items that can make you feel miserable in no small degree (think of sufficient carbohydrates, alcohol, added sugars, and hydrogenated fats).

Although all foods should be included in a balanced diet, you often just have to pause and concentrate on eating more nutritious food. This easy-to-follow clean-eat meal plan is a perfect way to get healthier food with 14 days of wholesome meals and snacks.

WEEK 1

Here's an alkaline diet schedule for seven days:

Day 1

- Breakfast: quinoa chia and strawberry

- Snack: an orange snack

- Lunch: salad sweet and savoury

- Snack: 1/2 cup of toast and dried fruit

- Dinner: plain green salad with olive oil and vinegar apple cider, 3-4 oz. Chicken roasted with sweet parsnips and potatoes.

Want to make the bubble of your focus, blast off the fat that you have accumulated in the wrong places, spring-clean your diet, turn the clock back on your skin, rock yourself and smash your insecurity?

Day 2

- Breakfast: great vegan apple.

- Snack: 1 bird.

- Dinner: salty wraps of avocado and stew of white bean

- Snack: 1 handful of pumpkin seeds toasted

- Dinner: plain cucumber salad with olive oil and vinegar of apple cider. 3-4 ounces. Brussels roasted chicken sprouts with red peppers

Day 3

- Breakfast: purple berry smoothie.

- Snack: 1 handle.

- Lunch: Noodles and Asian sesame

- Snack: a few dried apricot

- Dinner: 4 ounces. 1⁄2 baked sweet potatoes, beets curried and greens

Day 4

- Breakfast: Apple and almond butter oats

- Snack: 1 banana one banana

- Lunch: the cup of green goddess

- Snack: a few almonds

- Dinner: kale pesto courts.

Day 5

- Breakfast: smoothie strength

- Snack: a prosecutor.

- Lunch: Burrito quinoa dish.

- Snack: a few days

- Dinner: mushroom of wild rice, risotto of almond

Day 6

- Breakfast: chia pudding brunch.

- Snack: ½ cup of blueberry.

- Lunch: tofu-fermented miso soup

- Snack: a few macadamia noodles

- Dinner: roasted 4 oz salmon root vegetables

Day 7

- Breakfast: porridge quinoa.

- Snack: a few cantaloupe slices

- Lunch: Mexican salad. Lunch.

- Snack: a couple of slices of the dried cocoon

- Dinner: soup pumpkin.

Your wellbeing is a precious thing; take care of your body and mind so that you can live your lives to the fullest.

Diets are acceptable, but you will thank your body if you add an excellent workout to your balanced nutritional plan.

WEEK 2

How to plan your meal?

At the beginning of the week, a little planning goes a long way to making your week simple.

In this way, you can use the remaining chicken and quinoa throughout the week. Store chicken and quinoa leftovers in large glass meal preparation containers separately.

Day 1

Breakfast (338)

- 1 serving Vegetables Scrambled Eggs

Snack (119 calories) A.M. Snack

- 1/4 of a cup of hummus

- 1 cup cucumber sliced

Lunch (325 calories)

- 1 Veggie & Hummus Sandwich serving

Snack (30 calories) P.M. Snack

- 1 feather.

- 1 Greek Serving Kale Quinoa & Chicken Salad

Snack Evening (102 calories)

- 1 Broiled Mango serving

Totals daily: 58 g of protein, 1,216 calories, 121 g of carbohydrate, 60 g of fat, 26 g of carbohydrate, 1816 mg of sodium.

Day 2

Breakfast (307 calories)

- 2 cups Jason Mraz's Green Smoothie Advocate

Snack A.M. (35 calories)

- 1 clinic.

Lunch (328 calories)

- Mexican Coal Soup 1 1/2 cups.

- 1 cup of Black Bean Salad No-Cook.

Snack (92 calories) from P.M.

- 3/4 cup Kiwi & New Lime Zest Mango

Dinner (453 calories)

- 1 cup of cauliflower rice, heated

- 1 Soy-Lime Roasted Tofu Serving

- 2 cups of Colorful Pan Vegetables Roasted Layer

- 1 dc. Vinaigrette Lemon

Top riced colic with vegetables, tofu, and vinaigrette drizzle.

Daily Totals: 59 g of fat, 1.216 calories, 149 g of carbs, 44 g of protein,

42 g of fiber, 1,248 mg of sodium.

Day 3

Breakfast (290 kg)

- 1 serving Cinnamon toast butter-banana peanut

Snack from A.M. (64 calories)

- 1 cup of husks.

Lunch 370 calories)

- Chicken and Apple Kale wraps one serving

Snack from P.M. (92 calories)

- 1 feather.
- Eight mixtures.

Dinner (402 calories)

- 1 serving Asian Slaw Panko-Crusted Pork Chops

Daily Totals: 1.217 calories, 72 g protein, 127 g of carbon, 29 g of carbohydrate, 50 g of fat, 1.133 mg of sodium.

Day 4

Breakfast (270 calories)

- 1 Avocado-Egg Toast serving

Snack from A.M. (64 calories)

- 1 cup of husks.

Lunch (302 calories)

- 1 serving Greek Kale Quinoa & Chicken Salad

Snack from P.M. (95 calories)

- 1 medium apple.

Dinner (478 calories)

- 1 serving of Lemon-Garlic Butter Sauce Salmon & Asparagus.

- 1 Simple Quinoa cup.

Meal-Prep Tip: Prepare a hard-boiled egg this evening, so it's ready for P.M. Day 12 snack.

Daily total: 68 grams of protein, 1.209 calories, and 28 grams of fiber, 128 grams of carbohydrates, 50 g of fat, 1.233 g of sodium.

Day 5

Breakfast (290 calories)

- 1 serving Cinnamon Toast Peanut Butter-Banana

Snack from A.M. (96 calories)

- 1 clinic.
- 8 mammals.

Lunch (344 calories)

- 1 1/2 cup of Mexican cod soup.
- 2 cups of greens combined
- 1 dc. Vinaigrette Lemon
- 2 dc. Seeds of sunflower

Top with seeds of a sunflower.

snack (78 calories)

- 1 hard-boiled egg seasoned with salt and pepper

Dinner (408 calories)

- 1 serving Squash & Meatballs Spaghetti

Total daily: 60 g protein, 1,216 calories, 124 g carbohydrates, 56 grams of fat, 30 g of fiber, and 1,463 mg of sodium.

Day 6

Breakfast (264 calories)

- 1 cup of non-fat Greek plain yogurt.
- One-fourth cup of muesli

- 1/4 cup of blueberry

Lunch: (70 calories) A.M.

- 2 Clemens.

Dinner (325 calories)

- 1 Veggie & Hummus Sandwich Serving

- 1 serving Avocado Pesto & Shrimp Zucchini Noodles

Totals of 1200 calories, 68 g of protein, 133 g carbohydrates, 31 g of fibre, 52 g of fat, 1.102 mg of sodium.

Day 7

Breakfast (270 calories)

- 1 Avocado-Egg Toast serving

Snack from A.M. (70 calories)

- Two clementines.

Lunch (378 calories)

- Cucumber, tomato, white bean salad with basil vinaigrette 2 1/4

cup

- 1 slice of sprouted bread, toasted and 2 tbsp

- 1 feather.

Dinner (458 calories)

- 1 serving cocoon-shallot sauce fish

- 1/2 cup of Simple Cinema.

- 2 cups of 1 cup of mixed greens. Vinaigrette Lemon

Dailies: 1,207 calories, 113 grams of carbohydrates, 61 grams of protein, 60 grams of fat, 27 grams of fiber, 1 146 mg.

You made it!

Excellent job after this clean food programme. Whether or not you have made each and every recipe in this diet plan, we hope you find it inspiring, exciting and insightful.

The Alkaline Diet: A Powerful Weight Loss Plan

What if you knew that you're going to lose weight and feel younger? Do you want to try it? The alkaline diet and lifestyle have been around for more than 60 years, but many people do not know its normal, healthy and demonstrated weight loss properties!

The alkaline diet is not a fad or a gimmick. This is a safe and easy way to enjoy new fitness levels. You will find in this section what this dietary plan is, what makes it different and how it will yield results that will improve your lives and health.

Would you like to obtain a slender and beautiful body? If so, you are in the majority.

Sadly, more than 65 % of Americans are overweight or obese. When you are overweight, you possibly have ill health effects such as fatigue, swelling, sore joints and many other harmful health signs.

Worse still, you probably feel like you still love the body you desire and deserve. Maybe you've been told you're getting older, but that's not the reality. Don't buy into that lie. Don't buy into that lie. Other societies have fit, lean elderly people who enjoy good health in their 90s!

The fact is, your body is a beautifully built machine, and it is a good sign that the body is acidic if you encounter any signs of the malady. Your symptoms are just a call for assistance. This is for one day, and the body does not break down. Instead, your fitness erodes steadily over time and ends up being 'disappointed.'

What's wrong with how you eat now?

Normal American Diet (S.A.D.) concentrates on refined grains, alcohol, fats, meats and milk products. Both of these foods are incredibly acidic. In the meantime, we do not only consume enough of the alkalizing ingredients, such as fresh nuts, veggies, fruits, and legumes despite appeals from nutritional experts.

Briefly, our S.A.D. Lifestyle upsets our species' average acid-alkaline balance. Obesity, low-level aches and pains, cold and flu and influenza inevitably arise.

We lost our way. This is where an alkaline diet will lead to restoring our health.

• I'm sure you know the word pH, which refers to the acidity or alkalinity of something. Alkalinity is measured on a scale. You can take a quick and economical home test to see where your level of alkalinity falls and track it periodically.

• Medical experts and scientists have known this little known reality for at least 70 years. For optimum health and vitality, your body requires a certain amount of pH or the delicate balance of your body's acidified and alkaline levels.

And what does the correct pH balance and alkalinity matter to me? "These were concerns when I learned about alkaline feeding. You would think ..." I don't have to know all this chemistry.

We are going to use two examples of how acid and alkalinity play a part in your body.

1. We all know that there's acid in our stomach. This acid is necessary for conjunction with enzymes to divide food into elements that can be absorbed by the digestive tract. What if we had no acid in our bellies? Will we die of starvation because the body is unable to digest a slice of meat or something! Make sense?

2: Different body parts need varying acidity or alkalinity levels. Your blood, for example, requires a slightly higher alkaline level than your acids. What about your blood is too acidic? It will eat practically into your veins and arteries, resulting in significant internal bleeding!

While these examples show that the various sections or systems in the body need different pH levels, we need not worry about that.

If the body is long too acidic, many illnesses such as obesity, arthritis, loss of bone density, high blood pressure, heart disease and stroke may occur. The list is infinite because the body only gives up the fight for vitality and enters survival mode as long as it can.

A single alkaline diet.

Many diets rely on the same foods that first make you overweight or ill. You only need to eat less, eat throughout the day or mix them differently.

In fairness to the makers of this diet, they realize that many of us do not want to make drastic health changes. We want a diet based on processed and fried food, sugar, meat, alcohol and so on. Dietary designers just want to help us make improvements easier.

This is how we got used to feeding, and it's not just our fault! Greedy food manufacturing giants are keen to keep us eating like this. Profits in this food industry sector are much higher than in the processing of more basic foods such as fruits and veggies.

So, again, it's a different diet. If these other diets worked, you would not have to read this post, and you would feel lean, balanced and vital. You wouldn't need a change in your diet.

Here is a partial list of foods you should eat free of charge in an alkaline diet:

- Freshly made juices and Fresh fruits
- Fresh juices and veggies
- Cooked veggies
- Some soy and legumes
- Some eggs and Lean proteins
- Certain grains
- Healthy nuts and fats

You should eat these foods and beverages in small quantities:

- Dairy
- Many common grains
- Refined sugars and foods
- Caffeine and Alcohol

What is the alkaline diet like, and what can you expect?

Like any changes in diet or lifestyle, you will experience a period of adjustment. However, when you burn the cleanest fuel your body needs, unlike many food plans, you're never going to need to feel hungry. Moreover, once you are happy, you can eat all you want. You won't have to count calories, either. And you're going to enjoy a lot of variety, so you never get bored with food.

Consider an alkaline diet as a kind of 'fast juice' for the body. It's just not that serious. You eat nutrient-dense foods that your body longs for. If you supply all of the cells of your body that it needs so badly, the appetite goes.

Why do you suggest an alternative strategy such as an alkaline diet with all your diet plans out there?

When properly followed, you should expect the fat to melt more quickly than conventional plans. There are several testimonies that claim that people lose over two pounds every week. (And in most diet plans a lot of weight wouldn't be wise.) Plus your skin will get smoother, your stamina will improve, and you will feel younger.

Furthermore, the alkaline diet does two things that are essential to conventional diets.

1. It provides the cells with superior nourishment.

2. Naturally, it also helps to detoxify and purify cells.

This is why an alkaline diet works so quickly and safely behind these two truths.

One last notice when you consider an alkaline diet. Since it can be very different from the way you eat, you may wonder if you can return to your previous eating habits. The honest response is, it's clever to retain as many of the values as you can until you lose weight. But it doesn't have to be anything or nothing. Anything you do to follow a healthy diet improves the chances of weight well.

Seven Reasons to Go Alkaline and Avoid Acids

The body is a beautiful tool, with its many processes and systems linking each other to create a seamless machine that operates without problems. But, as with all devices, the body requires the correct form of fuel, and waste products get by burning this fuel are flushed out without any problems when they operate correctly.

Maybe once the body was perfectly healthy, and perhaps mankind once existed in a perfectly balanced environment, but we were unbalanced over the millennia; our diets and habitats were overwhelmed with acid and acidic residues. The issues associated with acidification vary from arthritis, fatigue, depression and even cancer.

Whereas not much can be done on global pollution levels, we can control our diets and what we allow in our bodies at least on an individual level. It may seem that it takes much time and energy to stick to an alkaline diet, but the advantages of going and remaining alkaline are well beyond the discomfort. There are hundreds of reasons for beginning an alkaline diet, but the top seven reasons for going alkaline to avoid acids are listed below.

1.) Loss of weight

This is a major one, so who didn't have a weight problem every time? And what would you have given for those who have to lose weight for an easy, safe and freeway?

The typical Western food and lifestyle are composed of many acidifying substances (refined meals, meat, sugars, and milk products) and habituates (alcohol, smoking and prescription medicines). And acids have a filthy way to consume and destroy healthy muscles, tissues and even species.

One of the body's automatic defence mechanisms is to generate fat cells to defend our fragile organs against these surplus acids. The purpose of fat cells is to eliminate this acid waste from the organs and store it in less significant areas of the body so when there is an abundance of acid in the body, the fat cells are bound defensively to the organs. Until these excess acids (thanks to a high-alkaline diet, proper hydration and exercise) are removed, fat cells are no longer required, and the body frees them from the task, resulting in weight loss.

2.) Enhanced energy

The other acids inside the body, the less the standard balance mechanisms of the body can function efficiently and the higher the body's acid levels. And the higher the acid levels, the more alkaline minerals (calcium, Phosphates, magnesium, etc.) are extracted from bones, tissues and muscles of the body to ensure that the blood can preserve the alkaline levels required to ensure that the body works. As the significant metabolism of these kinds of alkaline minerals is hindered, it contributes to leniency and fatigue. Leaching of minerals of this type was also associated with osteoporosis. As the levels of acid are decreased by proper diet and exercise, energy levels can rise.

3.) Allergy relief

An acidic environment converts the immune system into what is known as a "response mode," activating the immune system. The final result is that the body has an extremely enhanced sensitivity to everything; pollens, chemicals, etc. We know this increased sensitivity

as allergies. Any other ways in which the body is met with

unnecessary toxins and acidic waste is by soreness, swelling, eczema and excess mucus, all related to allergies. The allergies and their associated effects will vanish after excess acids are eliminated from the body.

4.) Return the Phase of aging

Aging is caused by a rise in acid waste and eventual decomposition of body functions. When the body is too acidic, and acidosis is present. Acidosis is essentially the tension of oxidation processes and the failure of lipids. Cells destroying cell walls and membranes are free radicals; destroy the cell walls and membranes before killing cells. As this happens, wrinkles, blurred vision, aged marks, faulty memory, tiredness, faulty hormones are visible; in short, premature aging. You can avoid further damage to your cells by eliminating these acids, and even reverse the breakdown process.

5.) Oxidizing

One of the side effects of acid waste build-up is that the cells of the body don't get enough oxygen, and that slows down the various functions of all cells. Much like the body itself, cells will die without enough oxygen. By removing the acids incorporated into your body, you will re-originate your blood by modifying your diet and consuming alkaline water.

6.) Blood Pressure Reduction

If a body is too acidic, cells tend to slow down their activity, and the heart has to work harder to compensate for their tranquilization, this induces high blood pressure. The addition of plaque to the arteries and the reduction in blood vessel diameter is another side effect of high acidity, which can also contribute to high blood pressure. By eliminating acid waste, you can enhance the functioning of your cells, and take some of the pressure away from your heart.

7.) Minimize opportunities for the development of degenerative diseases

In addition, almost all recognized degenerative diseases, including (but not limited to): directedness, osteoporosis, obesity, kidney diseases, liver disease, cardiovascular diseases, premature ageing, neurologic diseases, hormonal imbalances, and even many cancers, have been caused by the growth in body acid waste (or acidosis).

Degenerative diseases flourish in acidic conditions so that they can rob them of their ability to replicate or even take hold by eliminating their favorite environment.

What are you able to do?

If you really want to retain your wellbeing or to reverse any health problems, you should take one action right now and stick to an alkaline diet. You will take away the accumulated acid wastes of years by opting to consume all sorts of alkaline foods (fresh and raw salads, herbs, fruit alkaline, nuts, seeds) and drink alkaline waters.

The PH Diet Program To Weight Loss

If you are only trying to settle down before summer or would like to lose some serious weight, this plan will yield results for you – if you stay with it. You will ideally turn a 'diet' mentality into a 'lifestyle.' People become addicted to how you look and feel when you see the fantastic results of this program.

I won't guarantee you a pie-in-the-sky outcome. However, this software can quickly and safely make you lose weight. You will be fed well during the whole program, and that is why the weight comes off.

This program is not a complicated programme. You won't go through hunger cycles. In fact, you can eat much more often than average-only in smaller portions.

The pH Diet For Weight loss will turn your body into a furnace that burns everything you feed constantly and efficiently.

Why get your pH back to balance

As your body gets more and more acidic, it gets less effective. Acidification has a detrimental effect on metabolism and nutrient absorption. It slows down your metabolism and taxes all your body systems. Here are several ways that acidity helps to gain weight:

Stomach: mineral deficiency is associated with acidification. In a macro-mineral called chloride, the ability to absorb food in the stomach gets inhibited. For example, in order to digest protein food, your body uses chloride to generate hydrochloric acid (HCL). If you have chloride deficiency, the HCL formed by your stomach may not be acidic enough (i.e. your stomach is a very acidic organ). This leads to improper digestion and makes it harder for the rest of the digestive organs to repay.

Intestines: As the food is moved from the stomach into the small intestines, combined with bile from the liver and pancreas juices. These fluids must be alkaline to operate correctly. If the correct mineral balance is missing in your body, it can contribute to an acidic condition in the intestines. There is no proper digestion, no food ferments, and it putrefies in this setting. This ecosystem is a breeding ground for the development of all kinds of bad species. When these bacteria and yeasts proliferate, they literally boreholes in gut walls and leaky intestines. Now all this waste continues to make the whole body toxic. Around the same time, due to the lack of adequate digestion, essential nutrients are poorly assimilated.

Liver: This is the primary detox organ. With the acidity and contamination of your body, you put so much stress on your liver that it cannot literally keep up with the load. This stress leads to more stress on the other structures of the body.

All of this adds to the excessive fat

Fat is a toxin binder. This truth is well known, in fact, analyzed fat biopsies of more than 400 people, with disturbing results.

Each contained toxins (more than 100 different toxins have been identified). Imagine the scenario: microforms (harmful bacteria, fungi and yeasts), which include all kinds of toxins (mycotoxins and exotoxins) develop because of an acidic body. Your liver, already so overwhelmed from everyday activities, can't treat these toxins simply. There is also a lack of acidity and minerals required for the removal of toxins-not only is your liver too busy and heavy, but also not supplied with the requisite elements (minerals) to perform a very significant role.

Your body will deal with this issue in a beautiful way to store the toxins in your fat! However, since this fat essentially protects your life from toxins, your body won't allow it to happen, even though you have taken a crash diet. Furthermore, when your entire body is practically stressed out, your metabolism slows down considerably so that you store any additional calories that you do not need for fat. In the end, fat is a concern with toxins and toxins are an issue with acidity. If your whole biochemistry and pH are in order, you can actually see the excess weight melt away!

The Program

I will now describe a practical method of alkalizing your body, which will reduce your excess weight naturally. You will see unbelievable results if you stick to the procedure.

The purpose of the foods recommended is, of course, to obtain the nutrients recommended. If you are acidic, the nutrient forms that you lack vary from pH to pH. Proper pH equilibrium happens in your body when all nutrients are correctly synergised and abundant. These are the vital nutrients from the alkaline foods or supplements to help you control your PH and lose weight:

Water: This is the main ingredient your body requires. You have heard this your entire life, of course, but it's essential that you do what you heard. On top of that, when you want to clean out your entire system, I suggest that every 30 lbs of body weight, you drink one litre. So you must drink 5 litres of water a day during this program if you weigh 150 lbs. It not only serves to flush out acids and toxins from your body, it also helps regulate your appetite.

The consistency of the water you drink is just as important to remember as the number. You would want to drink heavily mineralized, alkaline water during this programme (and afterwards). This offers trace elements of essential value and serves as an acid buffer in your system. The cells of your body also retain this form of water better because of its composition. The addition of pH boosters to water would increase the pH to 500 times. It's a smart idea to manufacture one or two gallons at a time because when you want it, it's still readily available. Also, get used to taking you a bottle of water wherever you go. You can get water from consuming plenty of fresh vegetables as well as drinking water.

Trace minerals: these are the 70 plus forgotten minerals. They perform very particular body "niche" positions. Unfortunately, in the past century, a significant part of the soil where your food is produced lacks these essential trace minerals because of agricultural patterns. This initiative would help replenish these minerals' depleted reserves.

Alkaline minerals: sodium, potassium, calcium, manganese, magnesium and iron are included. The preservation of an adequate mineral balance is important for pH balance. When these minerals are in abundance, the body will be able to neutralize the body's excess acids and fluids.

Enzymes: Enzymes are life's spark plug. Life does not exist without them. Naturally, they are not cooked or stored in living foods. They are not only needed indigestion but literally millions of different chemical transactions in your body every day. Acidification means the failure of the enzyme. Each time you eat food which is fried, microwaved, refined or packaged, you eat food which is basically "dead." The enzymes in them that are essential to digest and assimilate nutrients are now gone. Anybody's organs are heavily taxed by the continuous consumption of these forms of food. High in fresh raw food, this program helps to replenish the essential proteins in your body.

And if you start using fat stores as a source of food, you would need enzymes (lipase) to bread solid fatty acids. This process would inevitably lead to excess pounds.

Fiber: In weight loss, fiber plays a vital role. Studies indicate that people who give their diet an additional 14 grams a day might expect to lose 4 pounds in weeks and reduce food intakes by as much as 10 per cent. You may not have much fiber in your current diet. The US average consumes 15 grams of fiber a day, 10 grams below the recommended minimum amount of 25 mg. This program raises the fiber intake well above the minimum RDA per day. It enhances the digestive process and gives you a "nice" feeling that will make you less eat.

The pH balance Diet

Your diet is mainly composed of: fruits, beans, noodles, nuts, fresh cold-pressed oils and powder of protein. These foods are alkalizing and moderately to highly acidifying for foods such as meat, milk, refined grain, sugar, canned food, cooked foods and more.

The diet is apparent. Eat at least six times a day, and maintain small portion sizes. Some call this kind of food "grazing." Many foods are low in calories (with the exception of oils). Yet calorie levels are not the answer to this dietary acid count. By eating these kinds of alkalizing foods, you introduce nutritional elements which help to neutralize and purge excess weight acids and toxins. You will also abstain from acidifying foods concurrently, so you will take a break to your body at the same time.

Shift your body

You don't have to get killed at the gym to enjoy the advantages of safe movement. The key is breathing and sweating. Have your heart rate up and pump your blood. You can significantly improve the benefits of this alkalizing diet and supplement program through daily exercise. However, not every exercise is the same.

It is much easier to keep the heart rate down for more extended periods than holding it high for a shorter time span. In general, when you work out, you shouldn't have to catch your breath, because the heart rate is too high. This would contribute to the burning of sugar as your source of fuel, compared with fat burning (which is what you want). It creates lactic acid in your body when you burn sugar-which, naturally, is not very pleasant if you cannot neutralize it efficiently.

This program is essential to make a lifestyle over time. When you hit your target weight, would you continue to keep it right? Do the same things that have succeeded you every day after this programme. The longer you are in optimum shape and the longer your body is in, the more likely you are to hold it up. The last thing, give yourself a back pat. You should be proud to take action to improve the quality of your health and your quality of life. Do not make this program a "chore" just have fun with it. Keep a smile on your face. Nothing – I mean nothing – feels as safe, dynamic, powerful and lean as a body. Nothing feels as safe as radiant! So go get it.

Chapter 3: Alkaline Diet Plan

Have you ever thought about today's diets and centuries ago, and how this could impact human health? Alkaline diet plan practitioners have been thinking about it and exploring the variations with some surprising suggestions for outcomes. In the past, people had a diet that matched acid with alkaline. It was only with the advent of agriculture and grain grinding mechanisms that people became more acidic and refined foods. Add salt, milk and sugar to this discovery, and you have a health catastrophe formula.

Acidic Diet Diseases

Many people claim that diets with high acidity contribute to many important diseases, including cancer, diabetes and obesity. Research to back up these arguments is not without critics, but there is proof that cancer cells in acidic conditions can grow faster. People who tried the alkaline diet plan swear by its efficacy. In addition, various doctors have suggested these types of diets for years.

Diet foods diet

A straightforward alkaline plan: tubers, nuts, legumes, vegetables, and citrus fruits. The secret to alkaline diet is just what you're not consuming. In order to obey the diet effectively, items like starches, sugar, highly processed foods, caffeine and alcohol, just to name the few need to be omitted.

Advantages

After you've been on your diet for a while, you'll find some changes in your feeling. Dieters also claim they have more energy than they had in years and show better skin, less weight loss or discomfort. The human body is fantastic and, when well fed, problems like cancer and other severe diseases can be prevented.

The medical profession has no faith in the alkaline diet. Doctors frequently deny the benefits claimed by advocates, but they would not caution against the alkaline diet if you have no medical reason to avoid it. Alkaline diet strategies are quickly accompanied by essential ingredients, so there are no complicated recipes or unusual ingredients. You won't find anything in the recommended food list not available from your local grocery; the most challenging thing is to miss the easy foods we're used to eating.

Lose Weight Fast

If you are among people who strive to lose weight, but who do not seem to win the battle of the bulges, it is time to allow the alkaline food plans to take over. You can change your life, lose undesired pounds, and get a balanced body with the right diet plan.

Crash Diet Weight Loss Plans Stop

Many people aspire to lose their weight by crash diet plans in the expectation that they can easily hit the perfect weight. Some dietary endorsers may also advise the use of diet pills to remove fat instantly. While dietary crash programs tend to work fast, they are often ineffectual and unhealthy.

Many that have turned to crash diet plans will quickly recover the weight they have lost. The reason for this? The majority of people who

have been eating for months will stick to an unhealthy diet once again. Failure to exercise is also probable that many people fail to maintain their ideal body weight.

A Permanent Solution Alkaline Diet Plans

Trying to find a successful weight loss strategy may be a massive challenge if you have a problem with being overweight. Yet a diet regimen provides a permanent alternative, called the Alkaline Diet Scheme. This particular dietary programme, which encourages healthy eating habits and a healthy lifestyle, is far from other crash diet programmes.

Bear in mind that what you eat directly affects your body. If you are not mindful of what you eat, your body will be loaded with toxins from the food which you eat every day. High acid content foods and drinks leave an acid residue in your body as well. The production of acid creates a chemical imbalance in our environment that can lead to obesity and even more severe diseases.

Conversely, the alkaline diet system focuses on holding the balance between acid and alkaline in our bodies. We will remove unnecessary acid and toxins from our bloodstream by taking the right food and living a safe lifestyle. The preservation of this balance is the secret to maintaining your ideal body weight in a tip shape.

Live Well and Prevent Sickness

Many people succeeded in their nutritional plans, and the most successful way is to adopt the alkaline diet. As we can see, this form of diet has healed some people with diseases like arthritis, cysts or even people with obesity and weakness.

Sickness is our life's greatest challenge. If a person doesn't feel well, he/she can't do the things he/she may want to do. He/she will not do anything to succeed, and he/she then turns to an unhealthy lifestyle.

The pH equilibrium needs to be maintained, and the average p H of the body fluids has to be 7,365 for our body to function correctly. Our body must also preserve an alkaline state instead of an acidic environment.

We need to remember specific items that can help in our alkaline diet plans:

Are you better aware of what an alkaline diet is?

It is exciting to know what the alkaline diet entails. We should note that an alkaline diet primarily includes fresh fruit and vegetables since they once metabolize alkaline residues in our bodies. Meats such as beef, pork and other dairy products are not alkaline and must therefore be eaten in minimum amounts.

Prepare ahead of time for your meals.

Planning your meals in advance is a healthy idea to completely respect your eating habits and sustain them. It is critical that you list the foods that are highly relevant. Although the first time you consume it, it is worth it because you have enough time to reflect and write down the foods which you can consume more, which will lead you to a healthier lifestyle.

Eat plenty of fruit and vegetables.

Since alkaline foods are mostly fruit and vegetables, you want to eat more. These foods have negative components that neutralize the acids that are positively charged when taken into our body.

The body retains a healthy PH status. There are also few acidic fruits and vegetables which are not recommended to be consumed in large quantities.

Know the PH balance value.

If we know the value of keeping a PH balance, we should concern ourselves with the kind of food we take. The liquids in our body have a healthy pH level to keep our body cells working well. It is not that we do not consume acid food at long last. In order to be healthy, 75%-80% of alkaline food and 20%-25% of acid foods must be destroyed.

Improving life takes little effort, but you can make a meaningful difference in your lifestyle with the right knowledge. It is only by alkaline diets that we need healthy eating habits.

Chart of Alkaline Food

Since at least 70 per cent for your alkaline diet plan must come from alkaline food, most of your vegetables can be consumed except pickled vegetables and sauerkraut. Base your alkaline diet on greens like wheatgrass, sprouts, kale, dandelion and barley grass.

Like beetroot, kohlrabi and radishes consume alkaline vegetables. Many fruits are alkaline and are among your best choices are ripe bananas, lime, avocado, lemon, cherries, and watermelon.

Reach chocolate, linens, olive oil and sesame oil for good fat. Olive oil, in particular, is filled with cardiovascular health-effective unsaturated and antioxidants fats, whereas flaxseed oil hold essential omega3 fatty acids which decrease inflammation and help brain function. Alkaline nuts, including almonds and pine nuts, will also make you healthy fat.

Choose whole grains such as buckwheat, kamut, spelt and millet and obtain alkaline-friendly lens proteins and carbs. Both mature seeds and edamame, white beans, soybeans, and lima beans, perform well in the alkaline diet menu. Other soy products, such as tofu, provide a source of alkaline protein.

Water hydrate and, if possible, grassy and green teas sweetened with an alkaline sweetener such as stevia. Bring flavour to your meals, including fennel, cumin, caraway and sesame seeds, using alkaline seasonings.

Alkaline diet Acidic Foods Restrict

If you adopt an alkaline Diet schedule, up to 30% of your daily dietary intake will come from acid-forming foods.

Limit processed grains like white bread, and select full-grain variants instead. Although whole wheat is still very acidic, it is the less acidic alternative than corn tortillas, white bread, or brown sourdough. Eat acidic fruits in a category that moderately contains pineapple, mandarins, raspberries, tangerine and unripe bananas.

Most meat is moderately acidic, with the most acidic being sardines, fish, tuna, beef, and veal. Dipping staples such as salmon, chicken, and freshwater also qualify as acidic food but are less acidic than beef. You would also have to restrict the consumption of milk products with the exception of alkaline buttermilk.

Do not cook with acid-forming oils such as butter, margarine, maize oil, and sunflower oils and cut acid-forming nuts like pistachios and peanuts. Minimize the use of particular condiments, such as mustard, ketchup, mayo and soy sauce.

Keep away from processed food; both canned and microwave foods are very acidic. You must also avoid acidic drink, such as cocktails of sugar-sweetened juice, beer, coffee, liquor and wine.

Menu Alkaline Diet

If you need a helpful description of what you can eat all day, here is a sample alkaline diet menu.

Alkaline solutions for breakfast

Start your day with a high-protein tofu scramble that is alkaline. Only crumble into pieces of bite, so it fits the feel of scratched eggs and adds your favourite alkalizing veggies.

For a spicier scramble, add steamed kale, mushrooms and a pinch of cayenne pepper, or try mustard greens, bok choy, and fresh ginger to make Asian-inspired dish featuring alkaline ingredients.

If you like to have breakfast with more carbohydrates, continue to cook millet with unsweetened almond milk to avoid burning to produce a balanced porridge. Add chopped almonds and sliced dried figs to your porridge, or add a sliced banana and a cinnamon dash to it.

Alkaline recipes for lunch and dinner

Using alkaline ingredients to prepare balanced lunches and dinners. Since leafy greens are among the most alkaline veggies, the alkaline meal is no brainer with a great green salad.

Attach a semi-cooked lens, a few blocks of tofu or a piece of barbequed chicken or salmon to your salad and make your good, spicy buttermilk with a combination of butter, olive oil, cayenne pepper and oregano. Top your greens with edamame, shredded carrots and baked chunks of tofu for Asian influenced salad, then make a dressing of sesame oil and fresh-grated ginger.

Make your favourite veggies a light, alkaline soup in a low-sodium vegetable bouillon, then toss them into edamame, sea vegetables and tempeh for high-quality protein and added flavour. Make a more hearty soup by adding a semi-cooked chamois or spelt pasta before serving.

Like Kamut, alkaline pasta may also fulfil a need for carbohydrates at dinner. Make the own alkaline pasta sauces home with food processor; make a tomato-friendly sauce made out of fresh basil, garlic and olive oil or a pure roast squash of buttermilk and sauge until fluffy

Serve on the bed of steamed greens with a white kidney bean, lentils and your favourite vegetables. Eat your chilli with a small part of grilled chicken or a slice of whole-wheat or germinated-grain bread, whether you are eager for extra carbs or protein.

Snack suggestions

Snacks can be accessible on an alkaline diet; have a ripe banana, a couple of slices of watermelon or an ounce of almonds. Try a quarter-avocado with a spoon of hulled sunflower seeds with a drop of honey when you seem to have more chance to plan your snack.

Or, mix an alkaline smoothie made from almond milk, a handful of chopped kale, a few frozen figs or bananas, and a spoonful of almond butter.

Hold the prospects

There are some possible advantages of the alkaline diet. Every day, you can typically eat plenty of alkaline fruit and vegetables that can reduce the risk of cardiovascular disease. You can emPHasize protein derived from plants over red meat, which can also improve heart health.

However, a large number of restricted foods in the alkaline diet can make it difficult to obey, mainly if some of your former dietary staples are classified as 'highly acidic.' Many acidic foods provide real health benefits; skinless chicken, for instance, is a rich source of protein and the supply of essential fibre and vitamin C by raspberries and pineapples.

Consult a food specialist to help you develop a meal plan which incorporates the fundamental concepts of the alkaline diet but still meets your individual food preferences if you are having a problem with the restrictions placed on the alkaline diet.

Alkaline Diet Recipes

Background detail about the alkaline diet and then a recipes, healthy blood was directly a result of a healthy or alkaline diet through his blood analysis. Foods were either alkalizing or acidic and when a person eats foods which mainly alkalize the entire body at an optimal level.

The Alkaline Diet Recipes are intended to alkalize the body, which consists solely of food alkalizing to the body.

The theory is that the fluid shape of these nutrients is more comfortable for the organism to assimilate. One of the alkaline dietary recipies is:

Green Smoothie Super Alkalizing

1 Cup of healthy water: alkaline water when available (naturally alkaline fresh spring water)

1 cup Bio Blueberries

Two big unripe bananas

2 pounds of spinach, dark or chard green leafy vegetables

Kelp, seaweed, dulse

One wheatgrass juice shot

Combine the ingredients with some ice cubes in a blender. Mix well and enjoy. A great start to your alkaline diet, this smoothie will overwhelm your day.

My absolute favourite is the next alkaline diet. It's effortless to produce and very delicious.

Salad Spring

- Spring organic salad mix
- Add some greens you're lying (horse, chard, spinach, collard)
- Currents
- Onions
- Olive oil
- Yellow Radishes Summer
- Throw the salad as you want and use it.
- New lemon juice squeezed.
- Spoon table sea salt
- Crushed dried oregano
- Crushed dried basil

You can change the quantities for the above recipe to your taste. The dressing tastes better if you can wait one day before using it. Both these alkaline nutritional recipes are very alkalising. The ingredients are really alkalizing.

Some still like to add newly germinated sprouts to their salads and other recipes. Sprouting is a simple and very inexpensive way of introducing super alkaline and biogenic food to your alkaline diet. Mung beans, broccoli and lentils are all excellent sprouting options. All you do is soak seeds overnight in a pot. Then you rinse and drain the seeds between 7 days 2-3 times a day. Keep the sprouts up until last day in a dark room or covered with NO sun. Then placed it in a position where moderate sunlight is obtainable for about six hours. You will find that when they begin to generate chloroPHyll, they turn green. Finally, add your favourite alkaline diet recipes to the sprouts and enjoy!

Top Alkaline Diet Recipes

Adopting a healthy diet is easy when you have access to alkaline dietary recipes To find at least ten recipes you want is really all you need to eat this way. Many individuals and families simply need just ten good recipes to turn from a regular American diet to an alkaline diet.

Alkaline dietary recipes can at first seem daunting because many rely on unfamiliar ingredients. Most people do not prepare tofu or other vegetarian forms of protein. There are also many strange alkaline vegetables.

However, at first, you don't have to think about that. There are also several alkaline diet recipes, including common foods. Only take the time to know which foods are alkaline and which foods are acidic.

How do you find alkaline diet foods to be enjoyed by your family? Start by scanning the list of alkaline foods and choosing which foods your family likes to eat. For you and for them it will be far easier to make a move with foods they know and enjoy already.

Build a list of recipes from the foods you already love and already know how to cook. As the alkaline diet recipes make you more relaxed, you can increase your range to include some more of the traditional ingredients. Many are shocked that they like kale or rhubarb or other "exotic" fruit and vegetables when they try.

Most of the bullying of alkaline food is that most people consume the vast majority of their nutrition from a cane or package. Since alkaline diet recipes are based on new, unprocessed food, when you are a recovering "fast food junkie," you will have to get ready for them. Cooking, like all skills, requires time to learn, but it is not impossible. After just a few weeks of cooking your own delicious, alkalizing food, you'll be shocked to do.

Where to Find Alkaline Diet Recipes?

The natural question is "Where will I find alkaline diet recipes when you first find out about alkaline diet and its many benefits-from great quantities of energy, vitality, its anti-aging properties, high digestion, preventing disease and generally boosting health?"

The refreshing response is that many recipes and foods you already know and love can be rendered alkaline by simply substituting alkaline foods.

The alkaline diet is followed by the exchange of acidic foods for alkaline food, such as milk, refined sugars and fats, meat, leafy vegetables, some nuts and fruits and seeds.

For example, the alkaline version of Bolognese spaghetti can be made by swapping hair from beef to brown lentils, swapping the Bologna canned tomato sauce jar for a homemade version with spices and herbs, tomatoes, some onions, flax oil and other unprocessed natural ingredients that are swapping hardened and together blended wheat spaghetti for raw Courgette noodle with Alkaline banana ice cream:

just have to take overripe bananas, peel them, break them into pieces and freeze them. When you like to eat ice cream, take ten or so chunks of the frozen chunk, combine them with some coconut or almond milk in your high-speed mixer, and a teaspoon of mica (a vegetable, a somewhat malt-like calciferous root meal), if needed. Also, you can add some lucuma powder or vanilla extract to make it 'creamy.' Easy, safe, savoury! It's hard to imagine there's no milk in this ice cream recipe and its consistency is just like the right ice cream.

As long as the fruit is consumed alone and in the sense of an overall vegetable diet before any other slow-digestion foods, they can complement it and help to alkalize your body. If not adequately mixed, it can ferment and cause acidification. It is also good to educate yourself of optimal food protocols.

A strict rule of thumb is to keep recipes as unprocessed as possible, raw and natural ingredients are the safest, and substitute fruits, beans, pulses, nuts and seeds with meat and milk products.

Some quick swaps help you to quickly alkalize your diet and body: coconut rice, milk, pasta and bread steamed vegetables; meat pulses; sugar processed fruits; coffee water and herbal teas, soda and alcohol.

Alkaline Diet Recipes Is Easier Than You Think

Do you try to find an alkaline diet?? It's not as complicated as you thought.

Adopting a healthy diet is easy when you have access to alkaline dietary recipes. Finding at least ten recipes you want is literally all you need to eat this way. Most people and families just need only ten good recipes to turn from a regular American diet to an alkaline diet.

Alkaline dietary recipes can at first seem daunting because many rely on unfamiliar ingredients. Most citizens are not used for cooking tofu or other vegetarian forms of protein. There are also several unknown alkalizing vegetables.

However, at first, you don't have to think about that. In reality, many alkaline diet recipes contain familiar foods. Only take the time to consider the alkalising foods and acidic foods.

How do you find alkaline nutritional recipes your family will enjoy? Start by scanning the list of alkaline foods and choosing what you consume your family's nourishment. For you and for them, it'll be far easier to make a move with the food you already know and love.

Create your list of recipes from the foods you already love and know how to prepare. With the alkaline diet recipes more comfortable, you can extend your range to include some of the more traditional ingredients. Many people are shocked that they enjoy rhubarb or other "exotic" fruits and vegetables when they try them.

A lot of intimidation is generated by the fact that most people consume the vast majority of their food from a box or a cup. Since alkaline dietary recipes depend on new, unprocessed foods, you must be used to them if you are a "fast-food junkie." Cooking takes time to learn like all skills, but it is not impossible. After only a few weeks of cooking your own delicious alkalizing food, you will be shocked by what you can achieve.

Chapter 4: How to Lose weight and Live a Healthier Lifestyle

Acid to alkaline diet is more spoken about today, but the majority of the population still do not know what it is. People who die early, have health issues, obesity, etc., usually have a very acidic internal atmosphere whereas people living at a very young age and who are not severely plagued with health problems have an internally more alkaline environment.

The majority of people are living in an impoverished lifestyle, consuming mostly garbage and unhealthy foods and continually exposed to other influences that have a dramatic detrimental effect on our wellbeing, as compared to acid and alkaline diets.

As a doctor myself, people always ask me what the best ways to stay well are. It is essential to pay attention to acid in alkaline diets if we are to live a safe lifestyle, not overweight, prevent severe illness and disease and generally live in right age with vigour and vitality. By studying your body pH and eating accordingly to ensure that your body is alkaline rather than acidic, people can experience things like fast loss of weight (by accelerated fat disposal), longer life, less stress, a more robust immune system, sleep stronger, more energy and may experience increased libido. Of course, these benefits alone are significant for wellness, longevity and happier life. By allowing the body to detox through the acid and alkaline diet, it is also possible for individuals to consume vitamins and minerals and to prevent many malignant diseases, including cancer and arthritis. Stress and strain on the internal organ are minimized with a more alkaline body, regenerating the skin, bones and cells and helping to keep you young.

In comparison, if the body of a person is too acidic, it can easily undergo obesity by accumulating and holding onto weight, ages faster, energy shortages are normal, diseases and viruses can be quickly and continuously established and an interior atmosphere in which yeasts and bacteria can easily flourish.

Many people in the West do not follow an acid-to-alkaline diet and are typically more acidic. This is primarily because of our diet. Consuming products such as processed food, burgers, fizzy drinks, a large intake of sugar, fried foods, unnatural fruit juice, processed food, energy drinks and transformed foods, all drive our bodies on acidic levels. Also, some foods that are otherwise nutritious are well known, such as strawberries, mangos and peaches, which develop an acidic environment in the body. Other surprises which also contribute to an increase in acidity include rice, salmon, oats and cheese, which means that these foods are limited by an alkaline acid diet. This is one reason why it is essential to know precisely what foods are producing an acid response and making you more alkaline. Other factors that make our bodies more acidic include different chemicals, tobacco, radiation, pesticides, artificial sweetener, air pollution, alcohol, narcotics and stress.

The optimum pH for all alkalinity benefits is 7.4. If your body takes 3-4 points, you're going to die! This is the pH scale:

0 = hydrochloric /acid total acid, battery acid

1 = vinegar

2 = gastric juices

3 = tomato, wine juice

4 = beer

5 = milk

6 = rain

7 = sea water

8 = pure water

9 = baking soda

10 = milk of magnesia, detergent

11 = lime water, ammonia

12 = lye

13 = bleach

14 = Sodium Hydroxide / Total Alkaline

The acid to the alkaline diet helps your body to stay at around 7.4pH. The reaction of the bodies to attempting to maintain this acid, alkaline balance is both unbelievable and fascinating. If the body is too acidic, it wants to make all alkaline. When this is done, the body retains some acid in your fat to prevent our body from damaging it, which is a positive thing, because then the body keeps on to the fat, so more weight is applied to it.

If there is excess acid internally, your body seeks alkaline in your bones and teeth elsewhere; however, your bones and teeth become so exhausted they become brittle and begin to decline. This can lead to many bone and teeth disorders, including arthritis and deterioration of the tooth. This is not possible if a person follows an alkaline acid diet.

Acid build-up naturally settles separately from your healthy organs but often gravitates towards your weakest organs already vulnerable to disease. It's like a bundle of wolves searching for the weakest of the pack and finding the simple prey. As the more fragile organs are targeted, severe problems, like cancer, can be detected much easier. It is necessary to note that cancer cells are sleeping if you are 7,4PH (which is the optimum PH of the bodies) and thus stress further the importance of keeping the acid-alkaline diet at a safe PH level in our bodies.

It also contaminates the bloodstream when there is the acid in the system. This prevents the blood from providing oxygen to the tissues. RBCs are surrounded by a negative burden so that they can bounce and travel very quickly in the blood and offer goodness.

However, they lose their negative burden when you are too acidic, and they stay together and travel very slowly. This makes them fail to supply our system with nutrients and oxygen. One of the first signs of this intoxication is that you tend to experience an energy deficit even though you sleep enough. It can be fixed very quickly by starting acid to an alkaline diet. This reaction is also caused by your blood after consuming alcohol.

Let us just keep this in context; around 33 glasses of water are required to neutralize one glass of coke.

One perfect way to make your body alkaline all the time is with green drinks regular. They are straightforward to produce, taste great and contain minerals, vitamins and chlorophyll that power our bodies. Chlorophyll is a significant part of the alkaline acid diet and green plant blood. It is a good blood builder, detoxification system, cleaner and oxygen booster. In fact, the advantages of chlorophyll are much too broad for this section. There are several recipes to make delicious green beverages.

Alkaline Foods - The 80/20 Acid-Alkaline Ratio

Many people like to eat so much that we fail to hold to the basics and reflect on our wellbeing. Without our wellbeing in line, we cannot always attain this ideal Physique, so it's still best to concentrate first on wellbeing.

Our standard way of concentrating on the outside and less on the inside threatens to destroy the majority of attempts for a bigger, leaner and healthier body. Of all the processes which are necessary for a Physical head-turning, the best thing for a well-functioning body is possible to lose out on your wellbeing at the cost of a temporary benefit.

To keep your body running at the highest level, you must ensure that all systems involved are not overloaded with toxins and frustrated by poor lifestyle choices.

Most of us don't live the right way, we consume incorrect food, we don't sleep enough, we're stressed out, and we don't get much fresh air. With the violence we get through, we can't expect it to operate as it should.

It's funny the way most of us get so upset when our bodies don't react how we want them to when it's just listening to what the body wants. Similar to a high-performance vehicle, power, maintenance and service must be provided sufficiently for the human body to ensure high performance and longevity. When we look after the body, the body takes care of the rest.

Today I want to explore the balance between acid and alkaline and how holding the right balance will help you improve your health, well-being and become slower.

The fundamentals first. Water has a pH (measured by hydrogen scale potential) of 7.0. This spectrum is known as neutral since water is neither alkaline nor acidic. Any pH-substance above 7.0 is alkaline, and any PH-substance below 7.0 is acidic. For a person, it is best to aim for a range between 6.0 and 6.8 to maintain a correct balance.

The acid-alkaline balance of blood must be stabilized by the food we consume and, as such, the body needs to be continuously supplied with potassium, sodium, magnesium, and calcium because these essential minerals contribute to neutralizing the acid waste accumulated through the ingestion of protein, sugar and starch.

Acid waste can also be incredibly harmful as it is known to cause a number of chronic diseases and health issues.

If you have chronic symptoms like water retention, migraine, low blood pressure, insomnia, sunken eyes, weak breath, acidic fruit sensitivity and/or alternative diarrhea and constipation, you may have acidosis. This word (acidosis) is possibly unbalanced and excessively acidic in your body chemistry.

Different changes within the body can also discard the average acid balance that can lead to an acidic increase in body fluids and to metabolic acidosis. Various diseases such as liver problems, stomach ulcers, kidney disease, obesity, anorexia, sugar disorders, fever and diabetes may rob your body of its natural alkaline base, but a low diet is usually the primary factor in creating an acidic body climate.

Note: Studies have shown that excess aspirin and vitamin C intake can also deplete the natural base of the alkaline.

When we work out to create a healthy Physique, we get too often enmeshed in protein and attempt to build up lean muscle that we are upsetting the body's average acid/alkaline balance and being excessively acidic.

It is difficult to practice and recover effectively when you suffer from irritating acidosis symptoms.

As I said before, proteins are acidic foods, and we need to consume alkaline foods to neutralize acid wastes from the intake of protein. This means that you can probably eat more vegetables than you usually eat with your chicken breast.

Seeking a perfect balance can initially be complicated and confusing, but it is the right way for an 80% alkaline and 20% acid ratio to be maintained. This means that you have to eat a diet which includes 80% alkaline food, and 20% acid food, to maintain a safe, balanced pH.

Proteins and starches are acidic, vegetables and fruit are alkaline. Almost all of the body's metabolic waste are acids, so we have to consume alkaline foods like fruit and vegetables to fall within the acceptable these acid waste.

Latest studies have shown that only about 15 to 20 per cent of fruits and vegetables are in the typical American diet. This implies that people in the country get the most of their calories from acidic foods. Given the current health crisis in America, I think it is secure to conclude that acidosis and disease are closely associated.

80% of your diet should consist of fruits and vegetables for optimum health. Starches and proteins should be the last 20%. This means that the diet is 80% alkaline and 20% acid.

This is a list identifying the foodstuffs alkaline and the foodstuffs acidic:

Alkaline Forming Foods

Vegetables:

- Broccoli
- Artichokes
- Cauliflower
- Cucumber
- Celery
- Cabbage
- Kudzu
- Mushrooms

- Spinach
- Green Beans
- Watercress
- Lettuce
- Onion
- Sprouts
- Radish
- Rutabagas

Fruits:

- Avocado
- Watermelon
- Coconut
- Banana

- Lemon
- Grapefruit
- Tomato

Nuts:

- Sesame
- Pumpkin
- Almonds
- Sunflower

Fats and Oils:

- Avocado
- Evening Primrose
- Borage
- Flax
- Hemp
- Olive

Acid Forming Foods:

- Alcohol
- Asparagus
- Aspirin and most drugs
- Beans
- Catsup
- Brussels Sprouts
- Cocoa
- Cornstarch
- Coffee
- Cranberries
- Eggs
- Most meats
- Flour based products
- Milk
- Olives
- Mustard
- Vinegar
- Pasta
- Sauerkraut
- Pepper
- Sugar
- Shellfish
- Soda, soft drinks
- Tobacco

Now that a specific food is acid-producing, it does not mean you can remove it from your diet entirely or avoid it for a long time. It actually does not mean that you can do it and just pick about 20% of your foods from the acid-forming food list. Most acid foods are also very healthy for you, except for a handful.

In the end, try as best as you can to abide by the 80/20 rule. As a result, your health and physical condition will significantly improve.

Train hard and look forward to the results.

Alkaline Foods List

The list of alkaline foods is more relevant than the list of emergency numbers. Create an alkaline list and paste it into your head and not only into your kitchen wall. The following time you shop for food, simply check the alkaline food list and shop accordingly.

Many plants and fruits are included in the alkaline food list. Cabbages, tomatoes, lettuce, shoots of bamboo, garlic, broccoli, germination, and nearly any vegetable is alkaline. Acidic, however, are dried beans, lentils and the white asparagus and must be avoided. Alkaline food list components should make up about 80% of our daily diet in order to maintain a similar ratio of alkaline and acidic ash in the body for optimum activity. There are various recipes to replace alkaline foods with acidic foods. Vegetables and fruit should be thoroughly washed so that raw fibers and alkaline ash can be consumed.

Most fruits are also on the alkaline food list except cranberries. Apples, bananas and citrus fruits are present in most areas at any time. In fact, melons and grapes are extraordinarily alkaline and should be eaten in abundance. As much as possible, fruit should be served to children because they are not only alkaline but also high-energy food that releases food. Bananas and apples are believed to speed up the treatment process since they are on the alkaline list of food and thus help the body heal more rapidly by the preservation of the alkaline body PH.

In addition to fruit and vegetables, dairy products are also included in the list of alkaline foods. Acidophilus milk, yogurt, buttermilk, and whey are all milk products on the alkaline table. Milk is alkaline, too, but just raw in shape. Both refined milk types are acidic and should not be eaten in significant amounts. For those who are able to consume non-vegetarian foods, no. If a protein consumption is to be made at all, then only specific proteins on the alkaline food list should specifically be adhere to. Chicken breast is healthy to eat and is safe to eat. All other meats, on the other hand, are all-acidic and do not form more than 20% of their diet.

Vegetables and alcohols are both acidic and not included in the list of alkaline foods. Yet herbal teas and coffee alternatives are also available to people who are prone to consume drinks. Herbal teas are retained on the list of alkaline foods and also safe for health. Honey is also a soothing food, and while children below one shouldn't be given sweetness, it's perfect for health afterwards.

Almonds, chestnuts and fresh cocoa are listed on the alkaline food list, while all other nuts are acidic. Quinoa and Amaranth are included in the alkaline food map and are also millet and buckwheat. Many other grains in nature are acidic.

The map of alkaline foods is a must to follow so that we can appreciate life fully.

Conclusion

If you consume an alkaline diet, you simply eat foods that are very close to what man should eat. You'll find a diet rich in fresh vegetables, fruit, nuts, legumes, and fish if you look at what we ate in our ancestors. Sadly, today's human diet is mostly filled with foods rich in unhealthy salt, fats, cholesterol and acidifying foods.

Even if some people assume that the diet of men has recently changed, the transformation from a predominantly alkaline diet to acidic diet probably started thousands of years ago. As soon as man began to cultivate his own food, things began to change. Grains have become a standard diet option, mainly since stone tools have been created. When cattle were domesticated, milk products and extra meat were added to the diet. Salt and sugar started to be added. The end result was a much better diet than many people are now consuming, but the transition from alkaline to acid began.

No trick, our western diet is made up of a large number of ingredients that are not safe for us. Too much junk food and "fast food" have our diet's consistency. The norm for obesity, along with an increased prevalence of diseases such as diabetes, cardiovascular disease and cancer, has become. If you wish to increase the health and reduce the risk of many diseases, an alkaline diet will contribute to returning your body to basics.

If food is consumed and digested, it causes an alkalizing or acidifying effect in the body. Some people become confused because the actual PH of the food itself is not related to the impact of the food when digested.

The body will become more alkaline instead of acid as alkaline foods are eaten. The blood PH can preferably range from 7.35 to 7.45. All healthy alkaline foods options

There are many advantages of changing the eating habits from acid to alkaline. It is less vulnerable to disease if the body is kept slightly alkaline. Most people have an increased energy level, anxiety and irritability, as soon as they start consuming more alkaline food. The development of mucus is decreased, and nasal irritation is minimized, making breathing easier. Allergies are also minimized by an alkaline diet. The body is, therefore, less prone to diseases like cancer and diabetes. Most people can only feel happier when they make a deliberate attempt to adopt an alkaline diet for a greater sense of health and wellbeing.